Ricardo the Rabbit and Friends

One of a Series Devoted to Correcting Speech Delays in Children

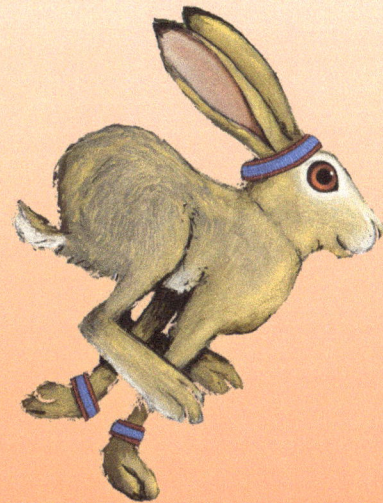

Praise for *Fiona the Frog and Friends*

"Drawing on personal experience with her own son, Erin Ondersma has written this book to address the needs of those with articulation errors. With vivid illustrations, a repeating text format, and many words addressing common childhood articulation errors, this book fills a need in children's literature. It offers several opportunities to practice target sounds and improve production. Speech/Language pathologists, teachers, parents, and children will find the book to be a helpful tool in mastering difficult to produce sounds."

—Erin Roon, M.A. CCC-SLP, Horizons DRC

"Speech sound disorders can impact up to 25% of children through age seven. We know from what research says that using auditory stimulation or "bombarding" children with targeted speech sounds can help improve their speech production (Wolfe et al, 2003). Through this beautifully book, Erin Ondersma has found a way to captivate children's attention and assist them with speech sounds that are frequently mispronounced. Enjoy reading this book with your child as you laugh and interact, knowing you are also providing a solid intervention for your child's speech development."

—Megan Hojnacki, M.A., CCC-SLP/L, Speech-Language Pathologist

Ricardo the Rabbit and Friends

ONE OF A SERIES DEVOTED TO CORRECTING SPEECH DELAYS IN CHILDREN

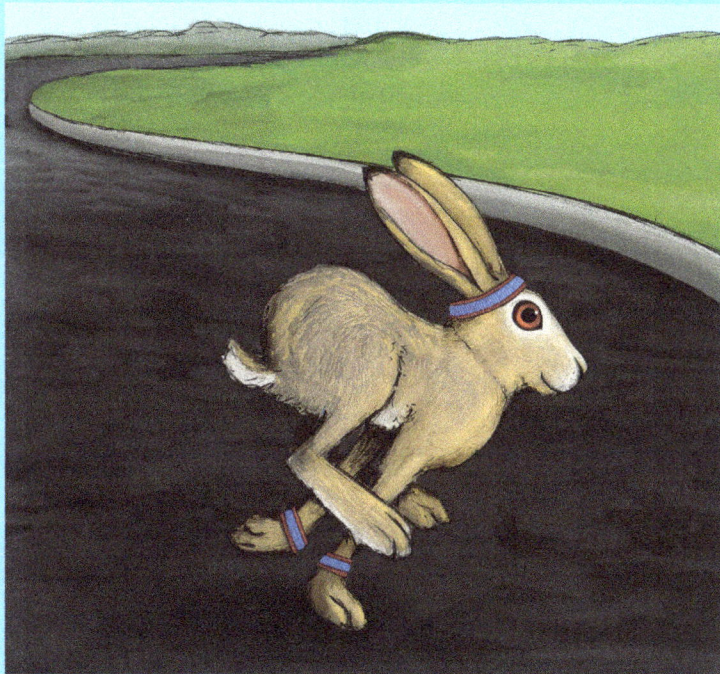

Erin Ondersma

Illustrated by Amanda S. R. Salazar

SUNSTONE PRESS

SANTA FE

Sunstone books may be purchased for educational, business, or sales promotional use. For information please write: Special Markets Department, Sunstone Press, P.O. Box 2321, Santa Fe, New Mexico 87504-2321.

Book and cover design › V. Ahl
Printed on acid-free paper
∞

Library of Congress Cataloging-in-Publication Data

Names: Ondersma, Erin, 1983- author. | Salazar, Amanda S. R., illustrator.
Title: Ricardo the rabbit and friends : one of a series devoted to
    correcting speech delays in children / Erin Ondersma ; illustrated by
    Amanda S.R. Salazar.
Description: Santa Fe : Sunstone Press, [2020] | Audience: Ages 8 |
    Audience: Grades 2-3 | Summary: "A book for children with speech delay
    issues where they read about characters running while learning to
    pronounce the letter "R.""- Provided by publisher.
Identifiers: LCCN 2020010034 | ISBN 9781632933010 (paperback)
Subjects: LCSH: Speech disorders in children--Juvenile literature.
Classification: LCC RJ496.S7 O565 2020 | DDC 618.92/855--dc23

LC record available at https://lccn.loc.gov/2020010034

WWW.SUNSTONEPRESS.COM
SUNSTONE PRESS / POST OFFICE BOX 2321 / SANTA FE, NM 87504-2321 /USA
(505) 988-4418 / FAX (505) 988-1025

For my niece, Caroline Hannah.

You are a thoughtful, creative, bookworm of a darling.
You remember all of the little details and know how to make us laugh.
May you always know how beautiful your smile is.

Preface

Dear Parents and Educators,

I began this series with my son, Hendrick in mind. Like many children, Hendrick struggles to produce a range of letter sounds and blends. He works with speech pathologists both at school and in therapy and we work together at home and at my daycare center on different exercises to help him. In my efforts to help my son with the sounds he struggles to produce, I asked his speech pathologists, "Are there books on the market that I could read with him at home and daycare to help improve his speech?" I was surprised that such books were not available and decided to write them myself.

My son used to be unable to pronounce the letter "f," which is why I began with the "F" book. Fiona the Frog and Friends focuses on several "f" sounds on each page. Shortly after Fiona the Frog and Friends came out, my son was able to perfect the "f" sound. He still is unable to produce the "r" sound, so I am eager for Ricardo the Rabbit and Friends to assist him with this commonly mispronounced letter. My nine-year-old niece, Caroline cannot produce the "r" sound either and I am super stoked to share this book with her!

My vision with this series was to create a fun tool, where children can enjoy the process of reading these books and taking in the fun illustrations without realizing they are doing "work." We have to do a lot of exercises at home and my son gets upset because these are things that distract him from doing the things he loves, like reading books or playing. So now instead of saying, "Let's work on your letter sounds," all I have to say is, "Let's read a book together!" His siblings cozy up and enjoy the story without realizing that the book is work for their brother. I really value inclusion in the day to day life of children with special needs and these books can be enjoyed by all children, whether they have speech delays or not.

There are times that my son has to be separated from his peers in order to work on trouble sounds. These books can be used at free play, in the reading corner, be read to the whole class, and be placed at audio stations. I want what's best for my son. I want him to master those problem sounds without being separated from the group. I hope your students and children will enjoy this book as much as Hendrick.

—Erin Ondersma

Ricardo the Rabbit
is running on the road.

Let's read together!

Can you say Ricardo?

Can you say Rabbit?

Can you say running?

Can you say road?

Let's try this!
Put your lips together like you are about to blow out the candles on your birthday cake!

Your lips should look like this:

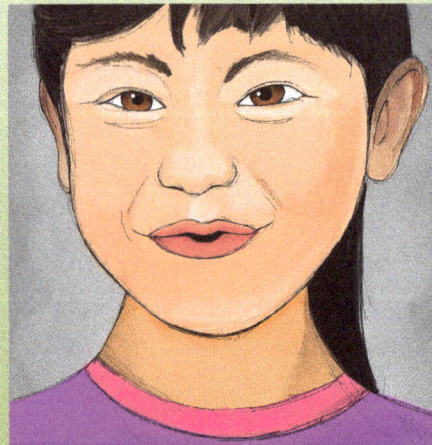

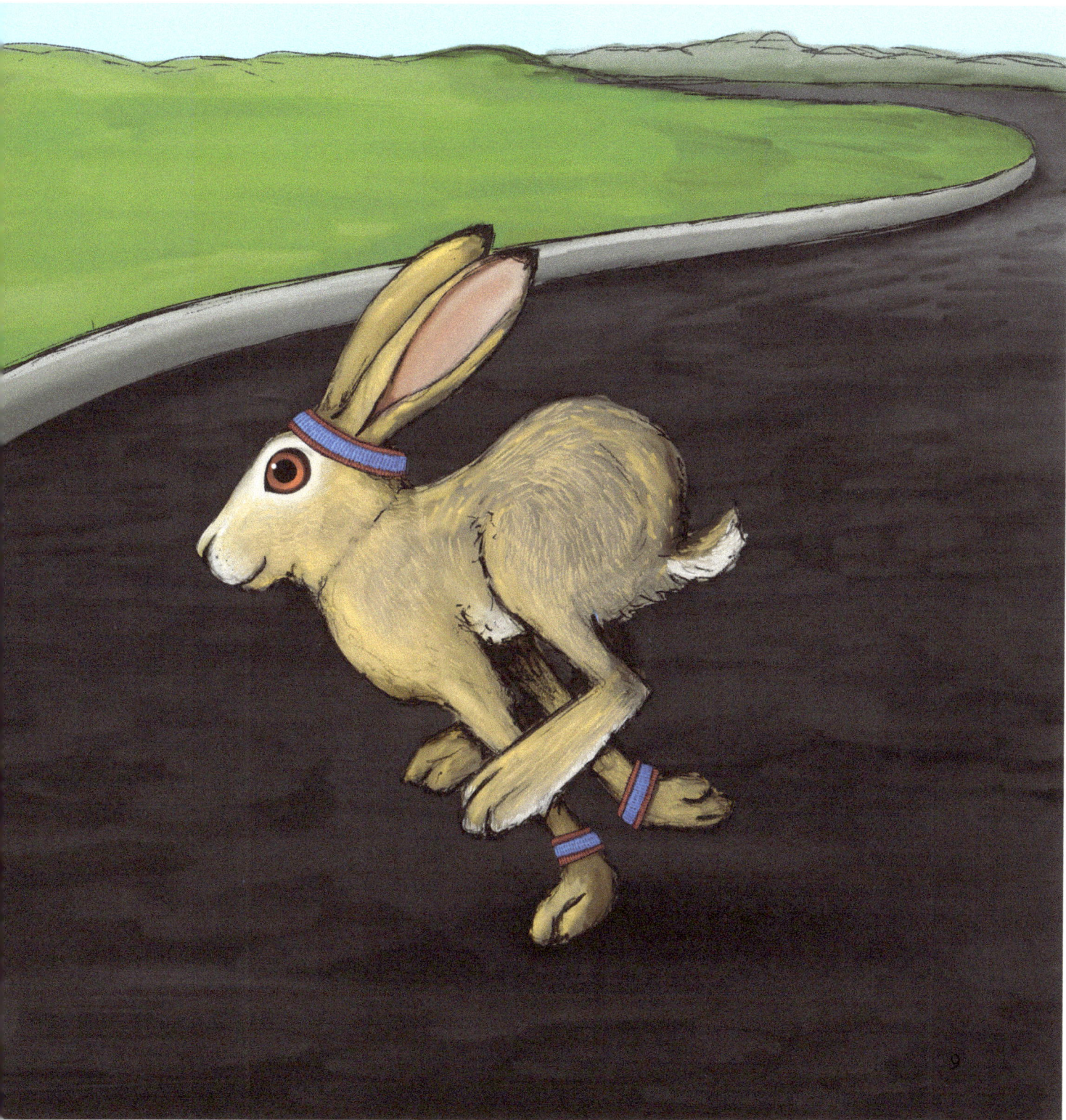

Rory the robot is running on the runway.

Now it's your turn!

Can you say Rory?

Can you say robot?

Can you say running?

Can you say runway?

With your lips pursed together like you are about to blow out a candle, place the middle of your tongue on the roof of your mouth.

Your tongue should be doing this:

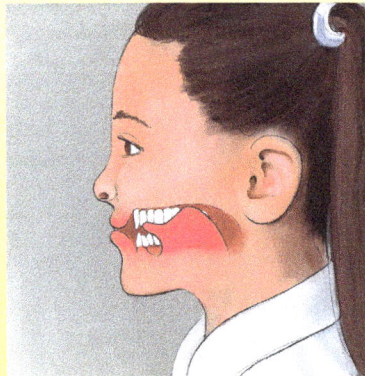

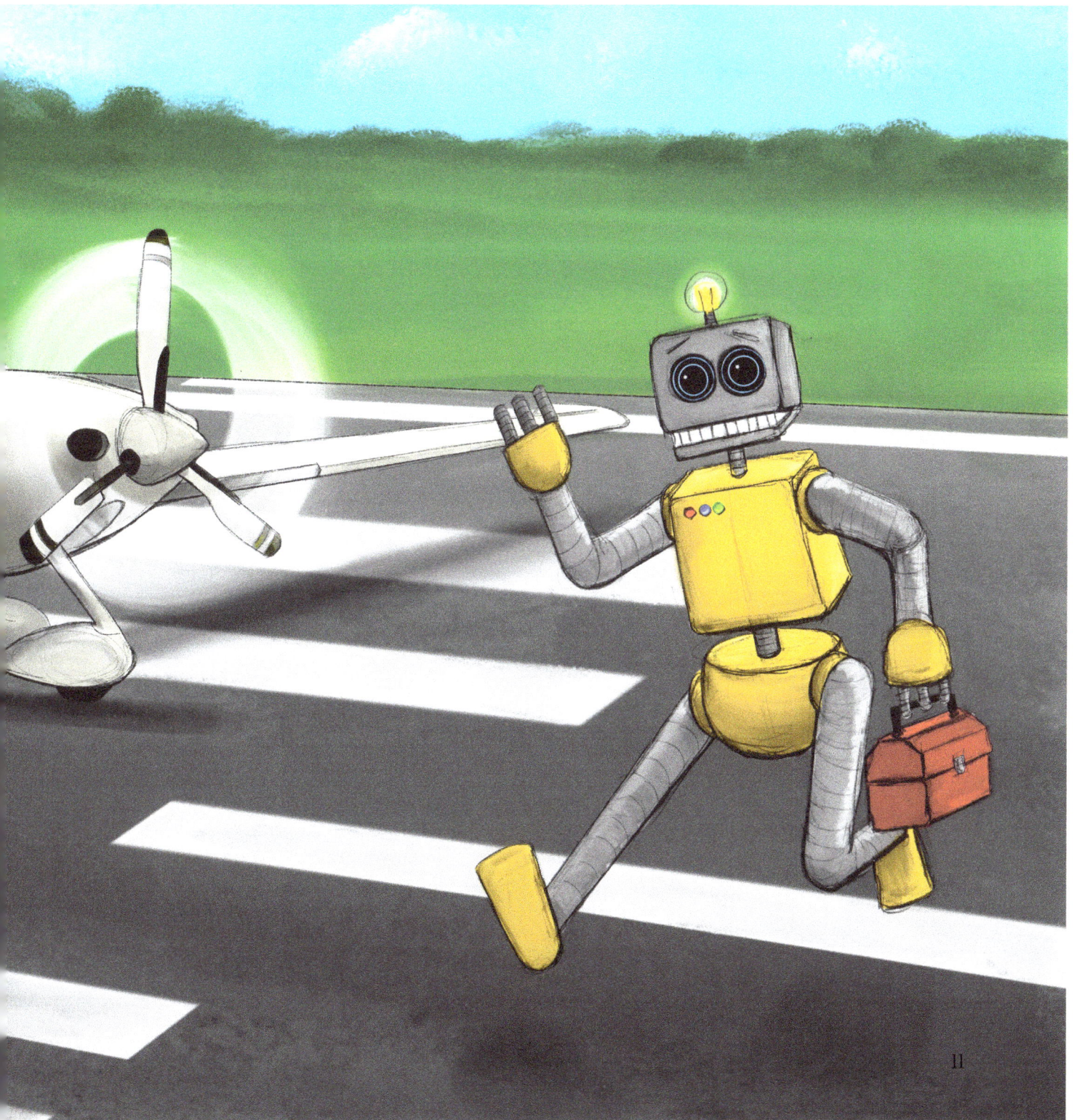

Rosa the robin is running on the rock.

Now you get to try!

Can you say Rosa?

Can you say robin?

Can you say running?

Can you say rock?

Grownup tip: make the "r" sound. Feel where your tongue goes when you make that sound. Place a little dab of peanut butter on the roof of your child's mouth where the tongue needs to land and instruct him or her to purse lips, curve tongue, and feel for the peanut butter. Reread the page together.

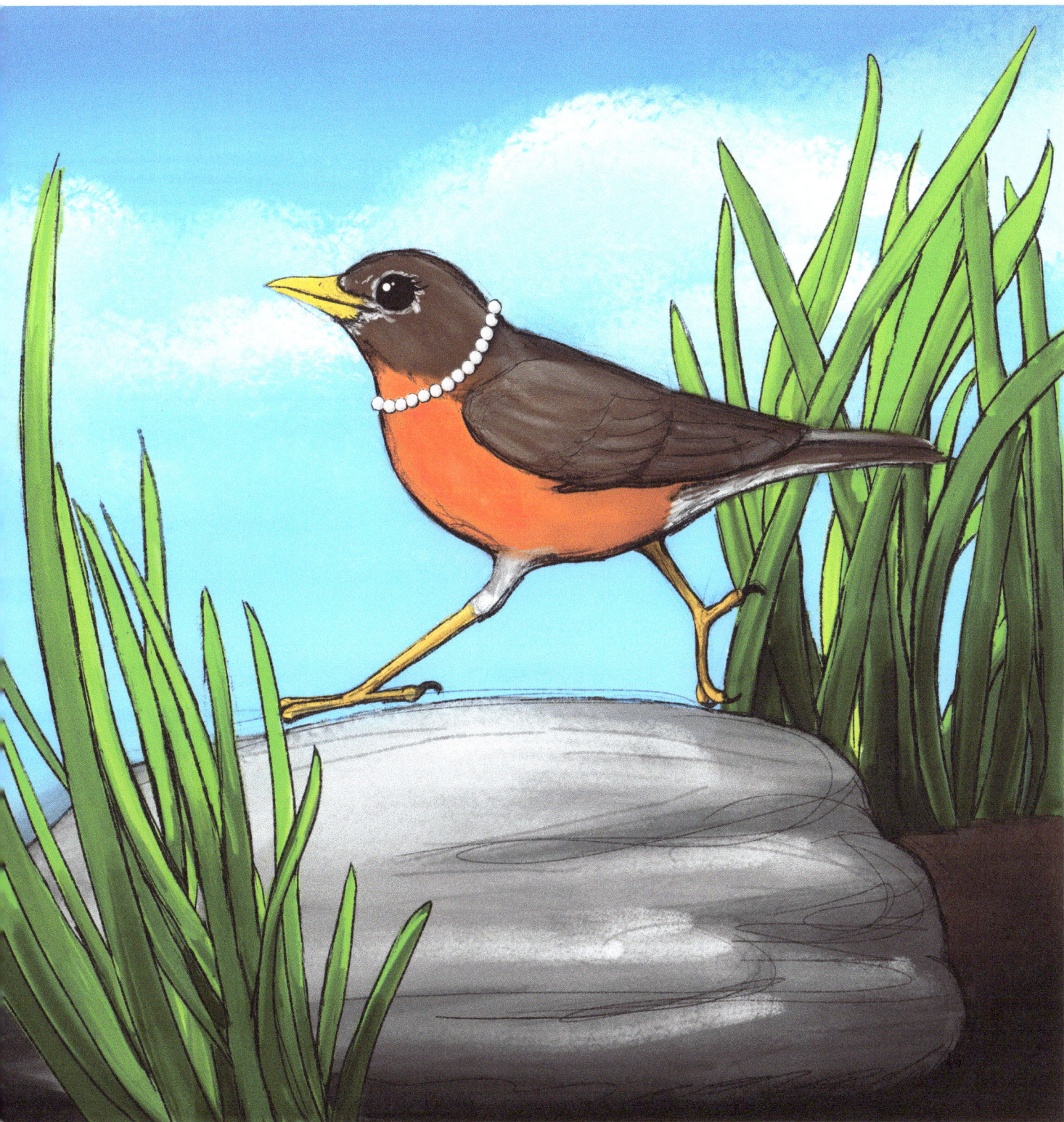

Rachel the reindeer is running on the roof.

You have a go!

Try saying Rachel!

Try saying Reindeer!

Try saying running!

Try saying roof!

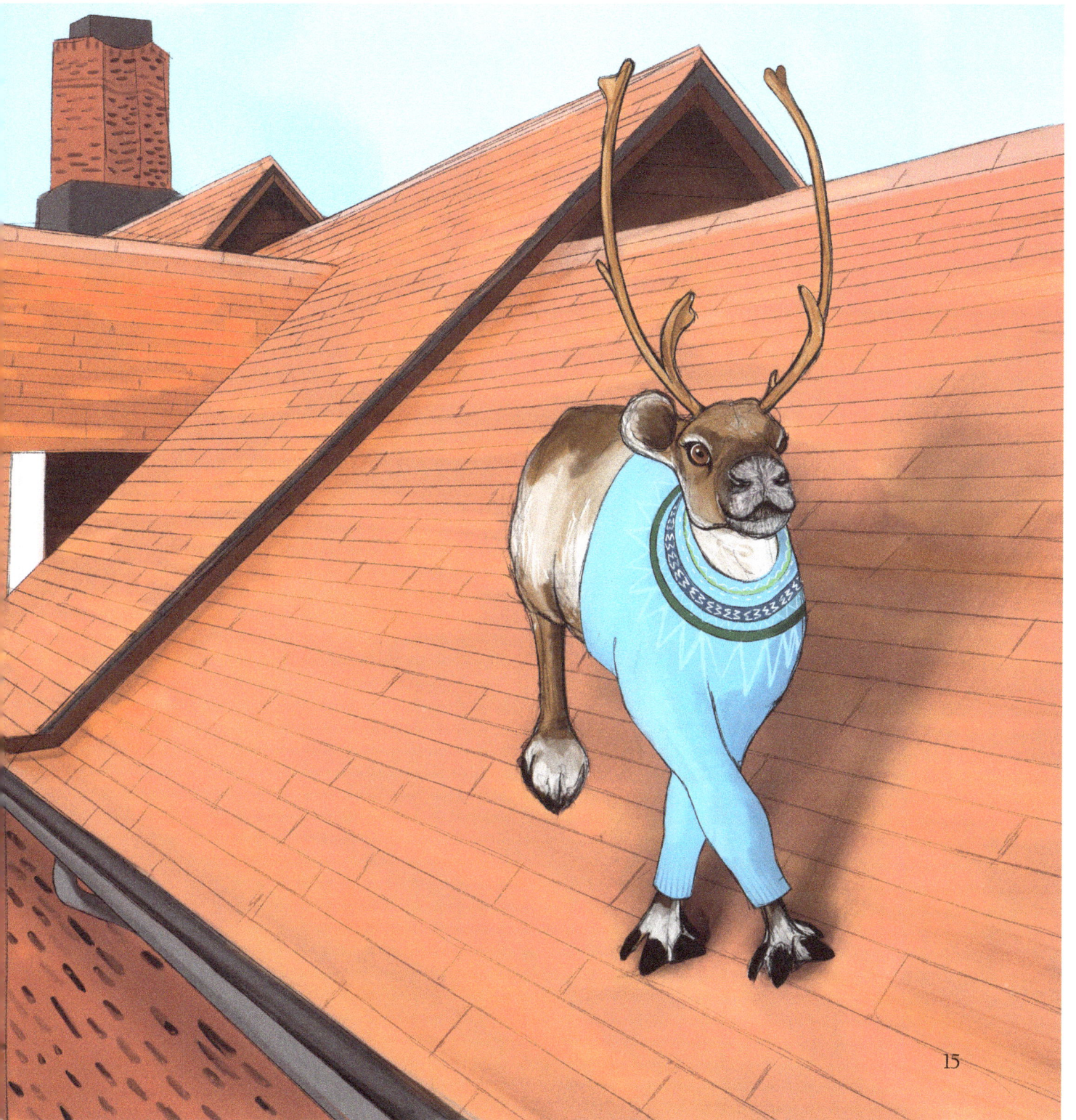

Raymond the rat is running on the rope.

Your turn!

Can you say Raymond?

Can you say rat?

Can you say running?

Can you say rope?

Do you remember how to put your lips?
Do you remember how to put your tongue?

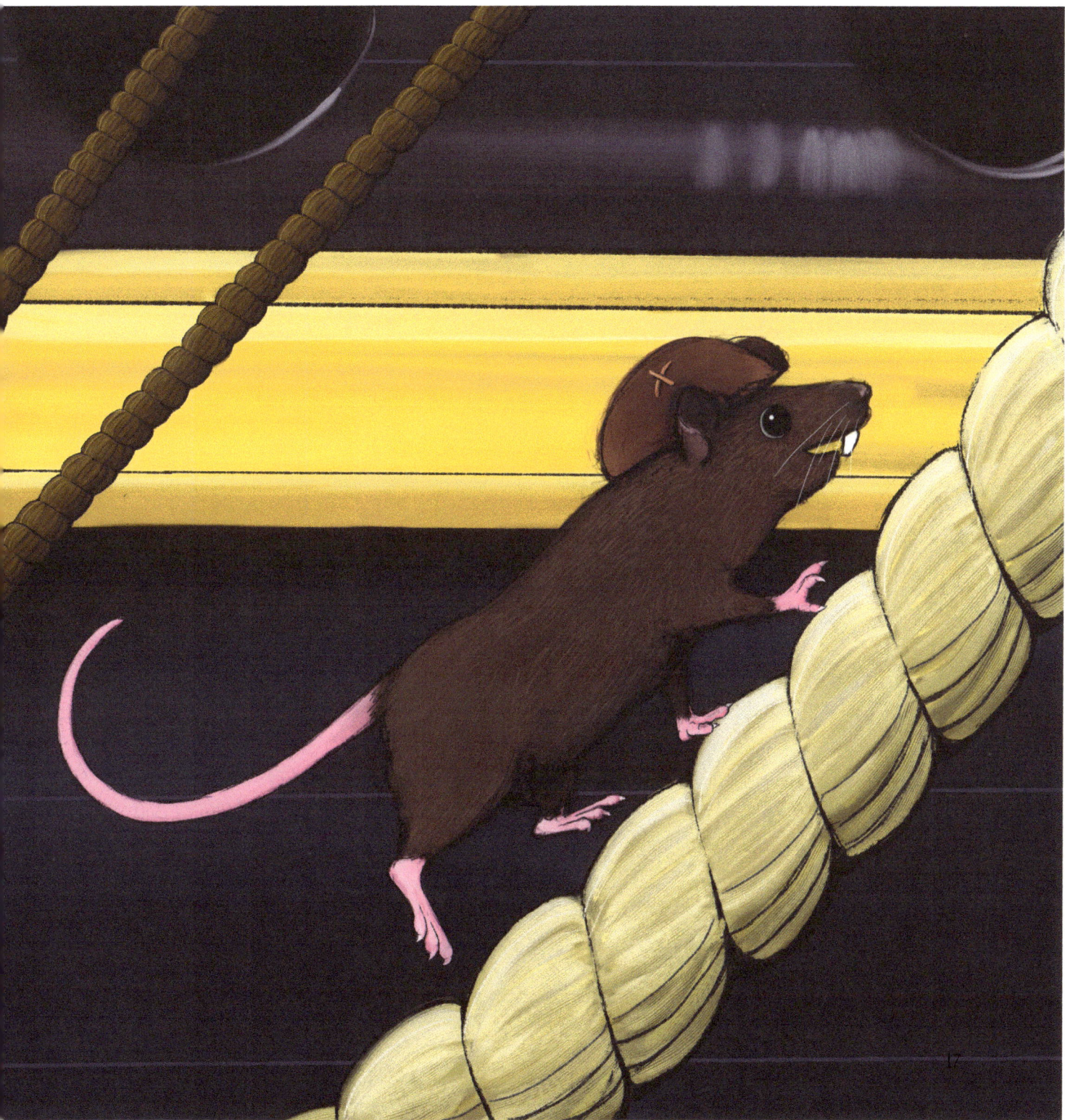

Ruthie the raccoon is running on the ribbon.

I want to hear you read this page!

Can you say Ruthie?

Can you say raccoon?

Can you say running?

Can you say ribbon?

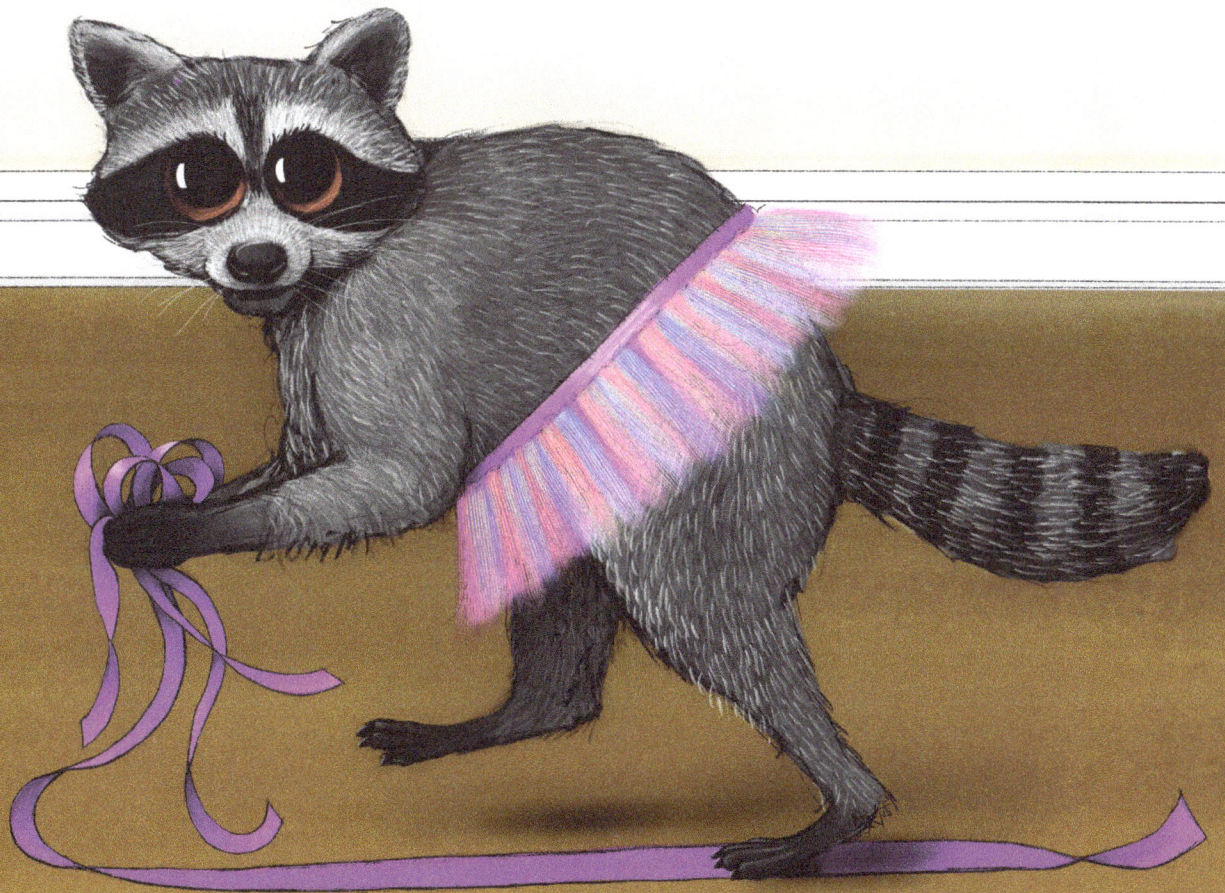

19

Rashida the rhinoceros
is running on the racetrack.

Let's do this together!

Can you say Rashida?

Can you say rhinoceros?

Can you say running?

Can you say racetrack?

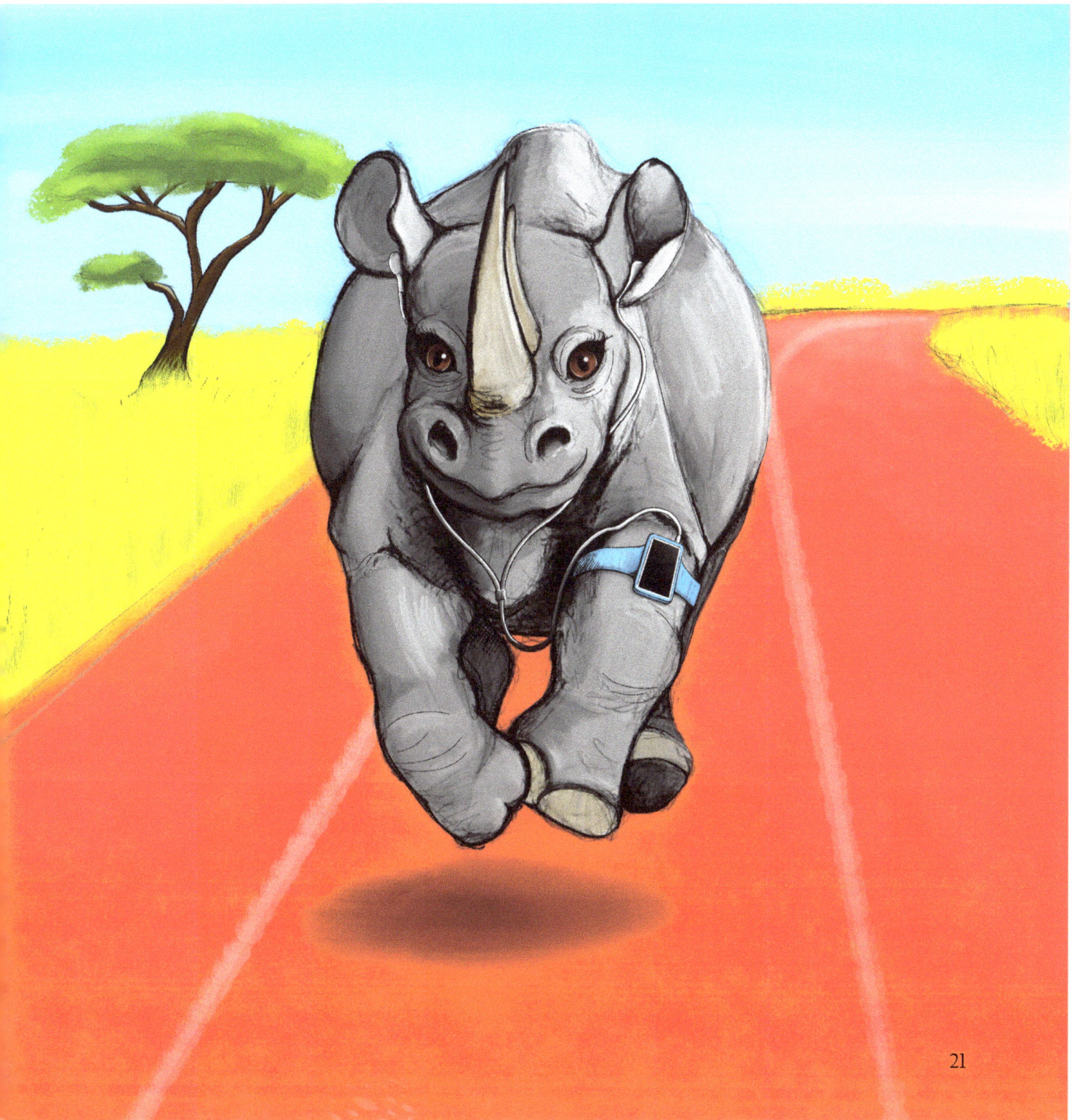

Randy the rooster is running on the rug.

Can you do it?

Let me hear you say Randy!

Let me hear you say rooster!

Let me hear you say running!

Let me hear you say rug!

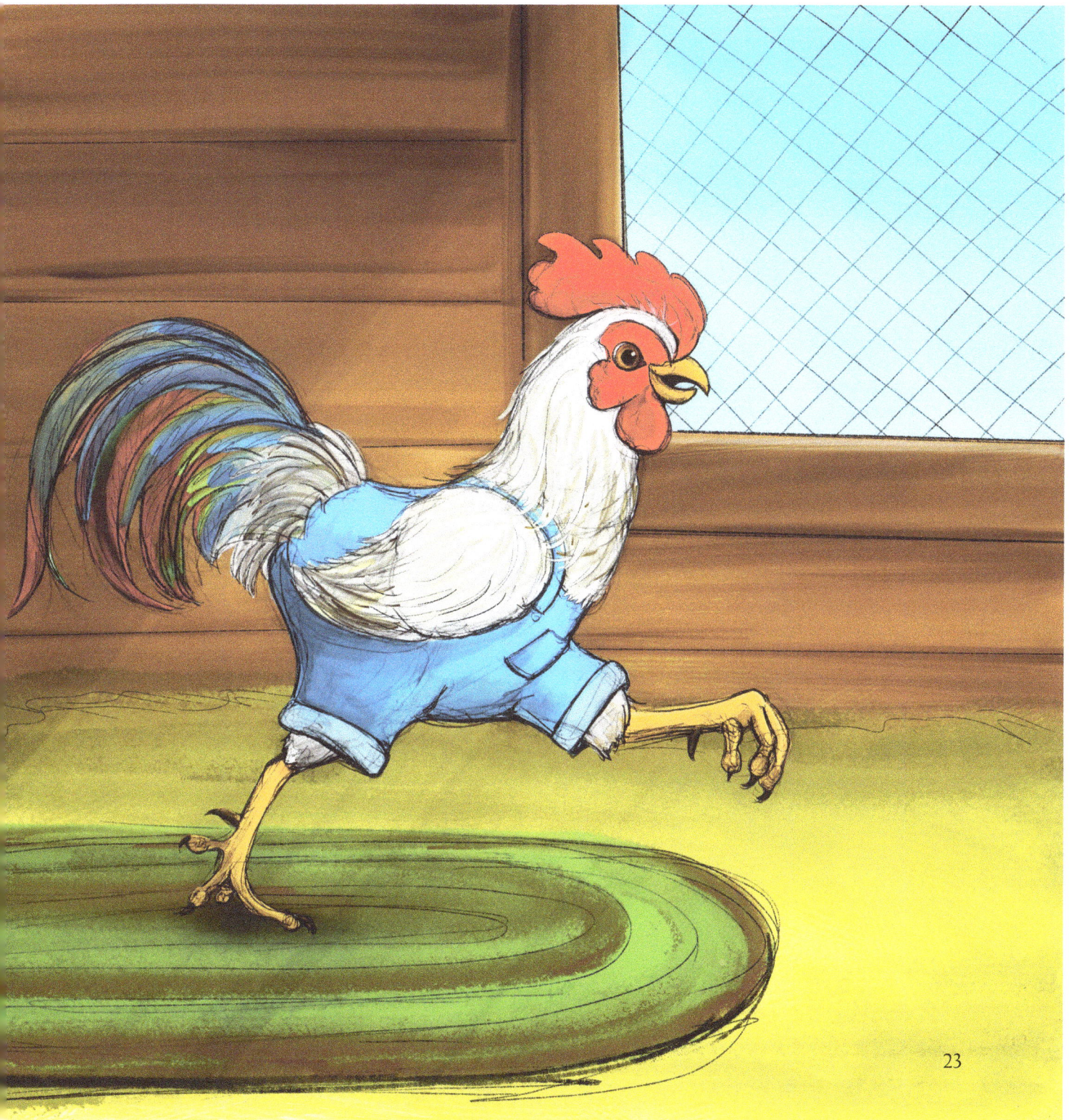

Reyes the raven is running on the reef.

I want to hear you try!

Can you say Reyes?

Can you say raven?

Can you say running?

Can you say reef?

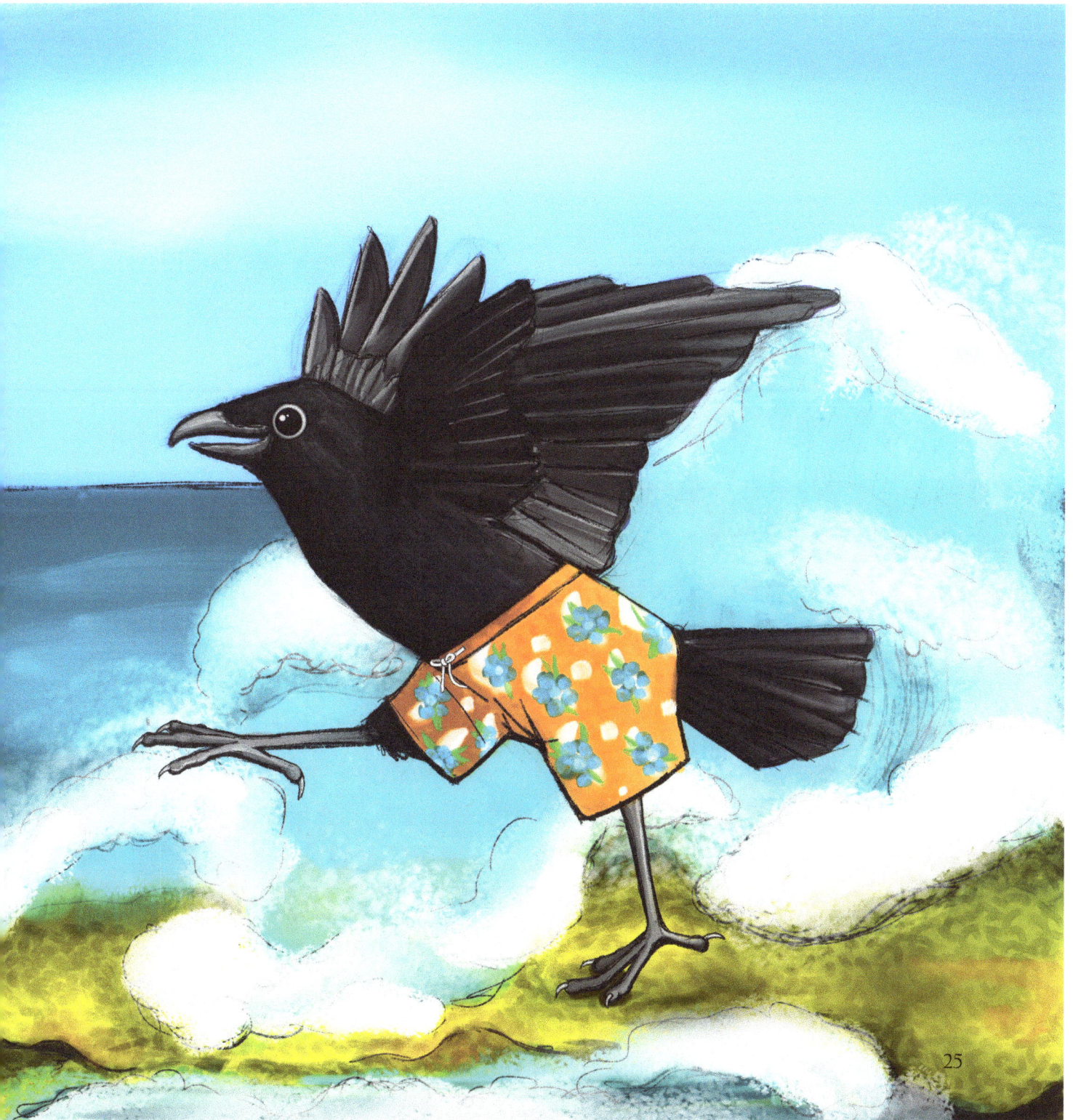

Roberto the rottweiler is running on the riverside.

Let's read together!

Can you say Roberto?

Can you say rottweiler?

Can you say running?

Can you say riverside?

Excellent!

The letter "r" is so tricky to pronounce! Keep up the hard work practicing. Practice may not always make perfect, but it will always make improvement!

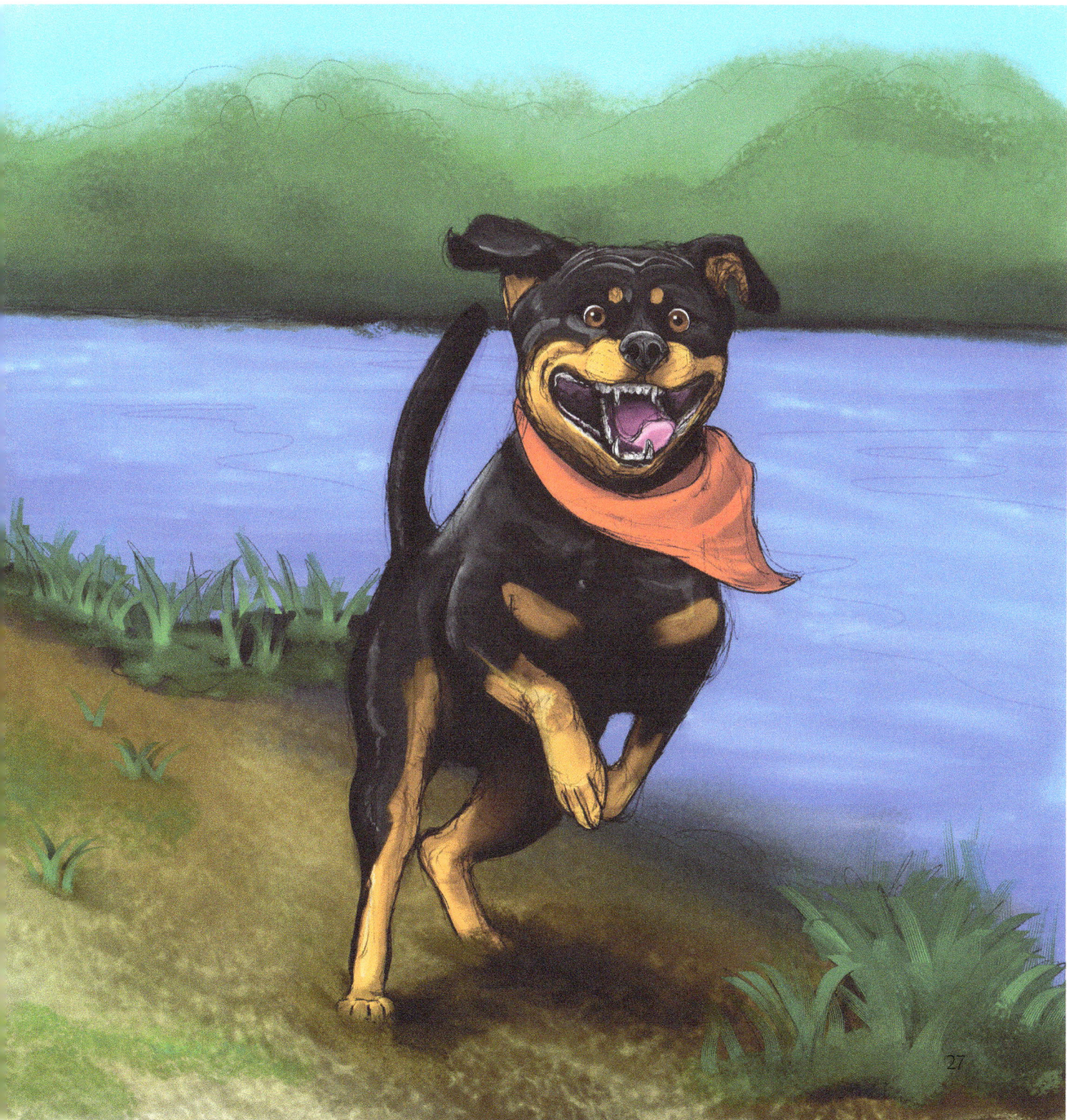

Other Information for Parents and Educators
(Information current at time of publication of this book)

From Barbara Levine Offenbacher, MS CCC-SLP, a New York State Licensed ASHA Certified speech and language clinician with thirty years of experience.

Excerpts from First Words: A Parent's Step-by-Step Guide to Helping a Child with Speech and Language Delays, Rowman & Littlefield Publishers, Inc.

For typically developing children, speech and language onset are automatic functions. Our challenge is when children are not developing or using speech and language within the expected window of opportunity, or when this delay or desire to communicate interferes with social language development and interpersonal connections. In the latter situation, the employment of a different approach is required, and according to the current literature, the earlier intervention is received, the more successful the result. You the parent are now empowered to intervene. You the parent now have a strategy to activate your child's innate process of communication, which for reasons that we do not fully understand is not emerging spontaneously. You will need to both encourage and stimulate your child's willingness and desire to communicate, while at the same time help your child discover language. Helping him integrate words and actions with meaning requires a strategy that follows the experiences of typical language planning. Now you have a fund of categories and words, representing a core concept of ideas, to facilitate your child's understanding about the world, and a way to prompt interpersonal connections, Your goal is to bring meaning to your child's confusing world.

The brain is a system of networks that are interconnected. These networks work in tandem, allowing us to process large amounts of simultaneous information usefully and effectively. To illustrate this idea, imagine you are sitting before a great symphony orchestra. With just the right timing, harmony, and loudness the conductor processes notes and instructions, which enables her to guide the many instruments, divided into five distinct groups, through a composition. Each member of the orchestra strives to play together as one, despite the fact that at times one hundred separate instruments make up the whole.

Our brain is that great symphony orchestra. The electroneural transmitters represent the notes, while different sections of our brain, referred to as lobes, represent the orchestra's instrument groups. The conductor, appropriately situated, represents the frontal lobe of our brain, the area I refer to as the captain of the ship. With the captain at the helm, the brain uniquely and amazingly blends a multitude of split-second messages, automatically, unleashing our human potential, the concert of all concerts. But what happens when the system fails? What happens when the uniquely human function of speech, language, and social communication fails?

For now, the diagnosis of a speech, language, and social disorder remains rudimentary, almost exclusively based on observation. The most overt characteristics are behavior outbursts, hypersensitivies, and at the core, speech-language delay. If you believe your child is delayed in language onset, research indicates the earlier the intervention, the better the outcome.

***

From Diane R. Paul, PhD, CCC-SLP, the director of Clinical Issues in Speech-Language Pathology at the American Speech-Language-Hearing Association.

Speech and Language Disorders
How to help your preschooler tackle the obstacles.
Reprinted with permission by PARENTGUIDE News and the author.

Effective communication is fundamental to human functioning. The development of communication skills begins in infancy, before the emergence of the first word. Any speech or language problem is likely to have a significant effect on a child's social and academic skills and behavior. The earlier the identification and treatment of a child's speech and language problems, the less likely they will persist or worsen. Early speech and language intervention can help children with reading and writing, in school and with interpersonal relationships.

What Is Speech?

Speech involves the production of sounds through the coordination of the breath, lips and tongue. Sounds form the basis of words used for communication. Some sounds develop earlier than others. For example, in English, children usually produce p, b, m, f, t and d before they pronounce s, th and r correctly. As children develop, they acquire the ability to produce more sounds and sound combinations clearly.

What Is Language?

Language differs from speech. It is a code in which we learn to communicate ideas and express our wants and needs. Reading, writing, understanding, speaking and some gesturing systems are all forms of language.

Language includes the meaning of words (semantics), the way words are ordered in a sentence (syntax) and the way messages vary depending on the listener and situation (pragmatics). For example, children learn to talk differently to an adult than they do to another child, or when they are in a classroom or on a playground. There are expected language behaviors for each age. However, children are individuals and may develop at different rates.

This is also true of bilingual children. They develop language skills just as other children do; however, every bilingual child is unique. Developing skills in two languages depends on the quality and amount of experience the child has using both languages.

What Causes Speech and Language Disorders?

Speech and language disorders may occur for various reasons including hearing loss, intellectual disabilities, brain injury, autism, Down syndrome, or other genetic or medical conditions. The disorders may exist from birth or result from an illness, accident or disease. The cause may be unknown. Speech and language disorders may occur together or separately and may vary in severity. Sometimes, the speech and language disorder is the primary problem; sometimes it is secondary to other conditions, such as autism or cerebral palsy.

What Are Types of Speech Disorders?

Speech disorders involve problems with articulation (pronunciation of sounds), fluency (stuttering) and/or voice (rough, hoarse or nasal voice quality). For example, children with articulation disorders may only be able to pronounce early developing sounds like p, b and m. They may mispronounce later developing sounds like r, s and l even in the later preschool years, and leave out sounds in words or substitute one sound for another (e.g., fum for thumb).

What are Types of Language Disorders?

Language disorders may involve speaking, listening, reading or writing. Some common ones for children in the preschool years include trouble understanding others (receptive language), making themselves understood (expressive language) or participating appropriately in social situations.

Children with receptive language problems may have difficulty understanding directions or questions, the meaning of word endings (such as not using "-s" for plurals, as in books, or not using "-ed" to indicate past tense, as in walked), or different types of words, such as prepositions, adjectives or questions. Also, they may not be able to follow a conversation or story, especially when a speaker talks fast or uses long sentences. In addition, they may misunderstand indirect or subtle requests (e.g., "It's a good idea to share") and only follow more direct instructions (e.g., "Give him the toy"). Furthermore, they may not pick up the meaning of gestures (such as shaking head or shrugging shoulders).

On the other hand, young children with expressive language problems may have limited vocabulary, use made-up words, leave off word endings (e.g., "-ing"), mix up words (e.g., remind and remember), leave out little words (e.g., the, and, is), use incorrect word order (e.g., "book me give") and use only short sentences. They also may have problems with social language, such as being too blunt or direct, changing topics abruptly, interrupting or not taking turns during conversation.

What Are Indicators of Speech and Language Disorders?

It is important to be familiar with typical speech and language developmental milestones. Here are some general indicators of speech and language disorders in preschool children:

Not crying to express different needs, responding to the human voice, or smiling or making pleasure sounds by 3 months.
Not babbling, vocalizing to toys or imitating some sounds by 6 months.
Not imitating gestures, imitating vocal quality of adult speech, understanding one-step directions or speaking a first word by 1 year.
Absence of any words by 18 months.
Absence of two-word phrases that have a message by 2 years.
Not using three-four word sentences by 3 years.
Echoing of speech after 3 years.
Poor intelligibility of speech (unclear speech) with familiar or unfamiliar listeners after 4 years.

Undeveloped play skills at any age.

Word-finding problems.

Dependence on gestures to follow directions.

Need for frequent repetitions of directions.

Poor social interaction with peers (does not get along with other children).

What Can Parents Do?

Parents can use various activities to help their child with his speech and language development. Here are some activities for preschool children (although specific ages are provided, most of the suggestions can be adapted and would be appropriate for children developing communication skills during the preschool years):

Children of any age:

Talk to your child about what you are doing, what you see, what your child is doing and what your child sees.

Repeat or expand on what your child says using correct sounds and words. Don't call attention to speech errors your child may have.

Ask your child to repeat or help with rephrasing if you don't understand what he says.

Take time to listen and respond to your child. Acknowledge, encourage and praise attempts to communicate.

Read to your child often. Describe the pictures, ask questions and talk about the way you read (e.g., turning pages, pointing out the words).

Use language tailored to your child's speech and language abilities.

Build and expand vocabulary by labeling and talking about objects and events in your child's environment.

Birth–2 years:

Respond to your child's early sounds and words (cooing, babbling, first words).

Imitate your child's vocalizations.

Use gestures to convey meaning and teach your child to imitate your actions (throwing kisses, clapping, waving, playing finger games).

Talk about ongoing activities (bathing, feeding, dressing).

Acknowledge and expand on the words your child uses.

It is okay to use a high pitched voice and "baby talk" on occasion to get your baby's attention.

Two to 4 years:

Repeat what your child says and indicate that you understand.
Help your child understand and ask questions.
Sing songs and recite rhymes to show the rhythm and pattern of speech.
Use photographs of familiar people and places and retell what happened or create new stories.

Four to 5 years:

Talk about spatial relationships (first, middle and last; right and left) and opposites (up and down; big and little).
Offer a description or clues and have your child identify what you are describing.
Work on forming and explaining categories (fruits, furniture, shapes).
Help your child follow multiple-part directions.
Follow your child's directions as she or he explains how to do something.
Play games and exchange roles.
Use television and movie time as an opportunity to interact and talk.

Who Can Help?

Speech-language pathologists are the professionals who assess and treat speech and language disorders. The American Speech-Language-Hearing Association (ASHA) can help you find a certified speech-language pathologist to help your child. Go to www.asha.org and click on "Find a professional." Or call (800) 638-8255 for a referral or for more information.

You may also call your local school to request an evaluation for children. A federal education law, the Individuals with Disabilities Education Improvement Act (IDEA) provides federal funding for individuals who need special education or related services, including those with speech and language disorders. Services are made available through the public school system.

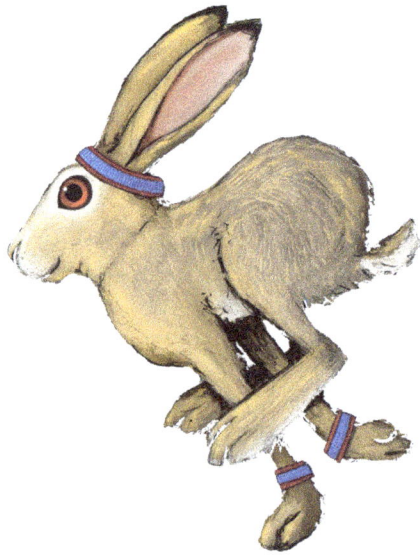

www.ingramcontent.com/pod-product-compliance
Lightning Source LLC
Chambersburg PA
CBHW041319290326
41931CB00045B/3500